CRYS

GW00869957

AND

GEMSTONES

Crystal types, their healing properties, how to care for them, and much more…

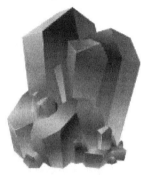

N JEFFREY

ISBN: 9798494591951

JOIN THE NIMPHLEEBOOKS MAILING LIST

You will be the first to learn about new releases, plus the many FREE and discounted Kindle books we offer!
https://tinyurl.com/NIMPHLEEBOOKS

DEDICATION

To the disbelievers, I hope this book has somehow enlightened you.

Also, to Michelle Lewis

CONTENTS

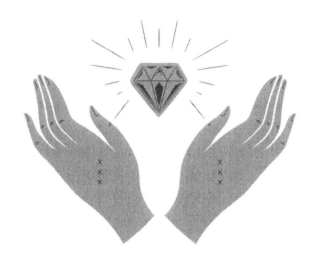

INTRODUCTION

Acupuncture, yoga, tai chi, and even healing crystals are examples of complementary therapies.

You've probably heard people talking about and flaunting these stunning stones. However, you may be unaware of what they may be able to offer you.

There are many different kinds of crystals, and some people believe that each one has its healing properties for the mind, body, and soul.

They are thought to promote the flow of good energy and aid in removing negative energy from the body and mind for physical and emotional benefits.

Aside from historical evidence of crystals being used in alternative medicines and rituals, astonishingly, there is no scientific evidence to support these claims. Modern science has proven the inverse: crystals do not work.

Yet, so many Crystals are marketed as ancient forms of medicine, with philosophies derived from Hinduism and Buddhism.

Nonetheless, earth's gift to humanity, crystals, have been used for healing and wellness for centuries. They are a powerful tool that can help you open your intuition and find a new balance in your life.

The information embedded in these rocks is manifested through their geometrical shapes and patterns. Crystals are metaphorically keys to our cosmic DNA. As they resonate with different frequencies, they resonate with the corresponding chakras. When placed in the correct position, they can enable more energy flow into the chakras related to the crystal's purpose.

Energy imbalances within us manifest as physical, emotional and mental disharmony. This can be caused by a dysfunctional relationship, unhealthy diet or lifestyle habit, a negative thought pattern, a traumatic experience or a long period of stress.

We may also feel oppressed by our bodies and mind. We need to learn how to work with these energies. We must find the profound meaning of these energies to heal ourselves and grow spiritually. When placed in its correct chakra, the energy released from the crystal will help you connect with your inner self and the earth. When the crystal is in its proper place, you will know how it can help you make healthy choices for your well-being.

The book you are about to read has been written with love and hope to help people connect with these crystal keys. I offer some simple crystal healing techniques for each chakra so that you can feel empowered through meditation, visualization and more. I hope that this book will improve your understanding about how crystals work in your body, mind, and spirit. Now it is time for me to share this gift with you!

CHAPTER ONE: THE BASICS OF CRYSTAL HEALING

It Starts with Energy

The Earth is a living, breathing organism. It is home to millions of animal species, other living beings, and humans. It plays an enormous role in the health of our planet and ourselves. The Earth's electromagnetic field is linked to human emotions because it taps into your body's electromagnetic field through the Earth's ground connection.

Your mind, body, and spirit work together to create a powerful energy system that is always available to use according to how you perceive your energy systems.

You are continually being affected by the energy around you without noticing it, because energy cannot be destroyed or created. It simply flows through things, travelling all around us. Its source is found at the center of the Earth. Our "field" of awareness is constantly changing as our feelings and thoughts fluctuate within this field.

We are all connected to the Earth's energy field and co-create with it. The more open we are, the better we will communicate with our inner power to heal our bodies, minds, and spirits. Everything in your body is influenced by how you feel emotionally.

These emotions create patterns that affect your physical body through your subtle energy system, which comprises energy fields (auras) surrounding your physical dimensional body (soul). We need to recognize that our inner potential is limitless. You can change your life because you can change your thoughts, feelings and emotions.

The earth's geometrical field has its unique energetic patterns. The geometrical earth field can express it through geometrical shapes, which are primary, secondary and tertiary forms. These shapes or patterns can be found in crystal healing or may appear during meditation or other types of spiritual practices. The geometrical shapes affect our energy fields, and the energy flows throughout the universe.

The earth's geometrical patterns can be recognized as crystal fields, which could be said to be a kind of geometrical poetry containing the language of symbols and numbers. These shapes can also come cloaked in energetic blocks, which need to be transformed and healed before the healing action is free to proceed. It is therefore essential to understand that we are all connected because we co-create this world together.

The incredible power of crystals is far less appreciated than their aesthetic beauty, despite their profound spiritual meaning. Crystals hold an infinite amount of knowledge about human existence.

What Are Crystals?

Crystals and stones carry and store particular high-frequency energies. They absorb and release energy the way we breathe in and breathe out. These stones have an energy signature that crystal stones can trace back to their origin. The "memory" of a crystal is stored within its molecular structure, which comprises atoms, molecules and crystals (ions).

Crystals are formed through growth atoms, which vibrate at a specific frequency that corresponds with molecular structure. Their geometrical patterns also determine how they respond to specific frequencies that match their molecular structure.

Crystal healing works because it releases old emotional baggage, negativity and stagnant energy from your body and spirit (energy field). The more we heal our bodies and minds, the more we will feel better and more balanced. Crystals help us reach a higher state of consciousness and access our spiritual power. Crystals also work on physical, emotional, and mental levels.

Crystals can be found in nature or made by human hands with remarkable precision. They make an enormous contribution to the planet's healing as they magically surround us with their magic energy fields. By working with crystals, you connect with a higher energy source that allows you to embrace a holistic approach to healing.

The Origin of Crystals

Crystals developed from minerals formed by the action of celestial bodies that came into being at certain times through natural processes over millions of years. They are formed when the elements are mixed in the correct proportions under the influence of cosmic forces. When this combination takes place, new features are created.

Crystals grew out of the earth's primordial rocks that were subsequently pushed up by movement in the earth's crust and then became exposed to heat, pressure and water. You can easily see how minerals form when you look closely at crystals. As they grow, crystals absorb everything they contact, including sunlight, water and various minerals in their environment.

Everything you see around you is made up of energy fields that carry information like the information found within crystals.

When the big bang took place, the universe was filled with energy. It then became shaped into self-contained forms that have their specific vibrations.

Crystal Grids

The Earth has a Crystalline Structure too.

There is a crystalline structure surrounding the Earth, which functions almost like an energy garment. The Earth's crystalline grid has been formed by the movement of cosmic forces and energy fields that have touched the Earth's surface over millions of years. It was created so that it can absorb and store information from other dimensions and field sources.

Crystals are present all over the planet in great numbers. The crystals on the surface of our world are aligned on certain latitude lines around the globe, thus creating a pattern on its surface called a "crystal grid." This grid is similar to an invisible spider's web covering almost all parts of our planet, including underground water veins that link to specific points on Earth's landmasses.

It is a grid that maintains and runs itself and is also alive and interconnected with all living things, including humans.

We can look at the crystals on the surface of our planet as a centripetal force—a force that holds together and draws things in as a magnet does. The physical crystal grid system of the Earth is like an antenna for receiving "information." It can comprehend vast amounts of information from other dimensions and store it in its internal dimension. It can send data to different extents, such as angels, fairies, foes, beings from other worlds and God's spirit.

Nature is our best example that we are not alone in this universe. There are other forms of intelligent life, and they are wiser than us. Not in the sense of age, in the sense of wisdom. I believe in the universal mind. It is the collective consciousness of all souls in this universe. All living things are part of the same consciousness system—whether animals, humans, trees or mountains, streams or rivers. We are all connected by an invisible thread that keeps us all interconnected.

Many people say we have an incredible connection to nature: You could call this a "sixth sense," but more accurately, it's called intuition— our inner guidance system. Our intuition is our best guide. It has many different functions, all of which are helpful to us. If we are sensitive, our intuition will give us the message.

Crystals & Chakras

The crystals on the surface of our planet are related to certain parts of our body, called chakras. There are seven of them that correspond to the seven colours of the rainbow—red, orange, yellow, green, blue, indigo, and violet. If your chakra is blocked, this will affect your life in one of two ways: either it will create physical problems or emotional issues. The chakras on the backside are connected with solar systems and universal forces on this planet. Your chakras are associated with all the entities in the universe, from angels to God's spirit.

Seven main chakras run from top to bottom inside our body, from the head down to the feet. The first chakra is located at the top of our head and is known as the crown chakra.

It is a connection between a person and universal energy—its function is to receive information from other dimensions, or it can even be a medium for healing other-dimensional beings. One of your main tasks is to maintain your ability to receive information from different sizes—this helps you in your daily life with every decision you make. If you forget this, then you will have difficulties with your life path.

The second chakra, which is located between the eyebrows, can be called a transformer chakra. This chakra has a big mission: to transform harmful energies into beneficial ones. This energy center has an extraordinary mission of protection from negative entities from other dimensions. Those who have been in contact with aliens have been implanted with crystals, usually, triangular which vibrate at a particular frequency—usually, this frequency is too high for us humans to perceive, but some people can still feel them.

The third chakra is located behind the ear, at the bottom of the middle part of the ear. It'd be called a solar plexus chakra. This chakra or energy center is related to our nervous system. It's related to our "little brain", which is below the cerebrum—the place where intuition comes from.

The solar plexus center has to do with our gut feeling. If your solar plexus guides you, you will know what's good for you or not, what's right or wrong for you, what you do or don't want to do in life.

The fourth chakra is located in the area of your heart. When you listen to the voice of your heart, you will be able to understand it and know what you want to do with your life. If this chakra is closed or blocked, you will not be able to understand your true feelings and will have difficulties in your life path.

The fifth chakra is located in your throat—this is a communication center, so if this chakra is blocked, you will have problems with speech and communication with other people.

A stomach chakra: The sixth energy center or chakra is located right above the stomach, just below the sternum bone. This chakra is one of the most important ones because it makes contact with cosmic forces.

It's connected with our solar plexus, our stomach muscles, and our throat chakra. If this chakra is blocked, you will have difficulties understanding your intuition.

The seventh chakra is located at the base of your spine, right above your sacrum bone—this is usually called a root chakra. The root chakra has a big mission: to be connected with everything that's happening on Earth. It's bound to all things happening on the Earth—with people, plants, animals and how everything lives here on Earth. This is also the reproductive center. It has to do with how crystals are created, your purpose and your mission on this planet.

The root chakra is connected to universal consciousness, the "big brain" of God's spirit. This chakra can be called a connector because everything created by God's heart passes through it to the Earth—the plants, animals, minerals, and humans. This energy center is connected to all things in this universe.

If any of your energy centers are blocked or closed, then you will not be able to connect with other dimensions, and you will not know God's spirit or universal consciousness.

You will also lose your sense of empathy; you will become numb and lose the ability to care about anybody else but yourself.

The crystals on our planet are related to these energy centers—they help us balance our energies, open our chakras, and obtain spiritual information from other dimensions.

How Crystals Bring About Change

Chakra healing is a clear and definite process. In contrast, crystal healing is a sophisticated and specific system that works with subtle energies that run through all life forms—it is a universal healing method rather than a local or localized one. Chakra healing uses crystals to balance the energy centers in our body, whereas crystal healing helps us to open the chakras and connect us with our spirit.

There is a clear difference between these two energy systems: chakra healing is used in a localized way—it can be done by one person or by a group of people, who will make the necessary connections outside themselves; in contrast, crystal healing uses crystals which already exist in nature and can be found in many types of stones and minerals, in food and even in water.

Crystal healing uses the method of frequency resonance—the energies of specific crystals are matched with the frequencies of the energy centers in our body. This is done through our intention, visualization or by using certain sounds or intonations. If this happens, then the crystal will begin to vibrate at a higher level. After this process starts, it creates a reaction inside the energy center connected with that crystal. The response will then bring about change in that specific chakra, thus healing any disturbances there.

Harmony is restored in our energetic system, balancing is made, and things will begin to fall into place. If you wish to heal your chakras on your own, this is quickly done through visualization, intention, and special breathing techniques.

The Importance of the Chakras

Our chakras are like little "energy centers" that are located in different parts of our bodies. They help us obtain energy from the Earth—this energy is what we need to give life to all our cells and hormones in our bodies. When all our chakras are open, we are healthy, well-balanced, and full of life.

25

Many reasons our chakra system may be affected—physical trauma, emotional traumas, or even spiritual shocks can cause them to close or become blocked. This will result in a decrease in energy levels in the body and the appearance of various diseases.

If your chakras are closed, it's usually due to fear caused by a lack of trust—whether this is related to yourself, other people, or God. When one or more energy centers are closed, there is a lack of openness within you, which will make it difficult to maintain relationships with others. You will also feel complete within yourself, which will prevent you from achieving many goals in your life.

You might also notice that the time it takes for you to heal is longer than usual. You will not be able to change anything until you open all chakras on your own—this is the only way to heal them and help them become balanced again. If this does not happen, then you may experience adverse health problems, including mental problems.

Another problem with closed chakras is that they may cause you to isolate yourself or even put up an emotional barrier between yourself and others—it could even be this way with God's spirit within you. If you are closed off, you will find it hard to connect with other people.

You may want to isolate yourself by withdrawing into your shell or even by closing off your awareness to others.

Opening the Chakras

The process of opening the chakras begins with your intention. You can do this by simply asking God or your spiritual guides to help you. Once the process of opening the chakras has already started, you will have access to universal consciousness—you will also have increased levels of intuition, creativity, and even new ways of thinking.

Opening the chakras will allow you to find new abilities in yourself—you will begin to receive information from other dimensions, and you will be able to connect this information with everything happening in this Universe.

This is also a critical step on your soul's path towards ascension because this process helps you connect with all your soul fragments located on different levels of existence.

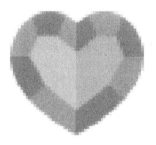

CHAPTER TWO: SHOPPING FOR CRYSTALS

This section of the book is about shopping for crystals—what are the different types of crystals that are available on Earth? What are some of the best types to use in healing and to connect with nature's spirit? There is also information about finding crystals—how does one do this? And how do we know if a crystal is authentic or not.

Types of Healing crystals

There are many different types of healing crystals. The three most common and useful for healing and spiritual work are Quartz, Amethyst, and tourmaline. Quartz is fine-grained and usually transparent or rose-colored. Some quartz is black, but it all has the same healing properties. Amethyst is purple Quartz and is also a potent healing tool for spiritual work and physical ailments such as depression, headaches, blood problems, menstrual cramps and even some heart problems.

1. Clear Quartz

This is the "master healer" crystal and is probably the most common. This type of Quartz is transparent with a waxy luster. It enhances the immune system and can be paired with other crystals to amplify its effects. It is used for healing, meditation, connection with the divine, clarity of mind, intuition, psychic powers, energy work and harmonizing with Mother Earth.

2. Rose Quartz

This crystal has a very noticeable pink to a reddish hue and is also used for healing and connecting with the divine feminine energy, or God as a woman. Rose quartz, we can use this type of crystal for healing broken hearts and acts as a calming agent, but quartz can also be used to give energy to those who have been traumatized or have had major surgery. It is also used to protect from negative energies from those who wish to harm or cause trouble in one's life.

3. Amethyst

This crystal is purple Quartz which is considered one of the most powerful crystals in the world because of its strong connection with the divine feminine. This is an excellent crystal for spiritual teachers, healers and anyone who wishes to connect or communicate with their higher self or God or Goddess.

4. Jasper

Jasper is a powerfully grounding crystal which acts quickly to heal and balance the chakras. It has a pronounced purple color and can be used to help release old patterns and open the aura for spiritual growth.

5. Lavender Quartz

This crystal is another form of rose quartz because it also comes in rose color but is extremely powerful in its own right because it makes sense with the natural flow of life and growth, acting as a gentle cleanser for all things that need to grow and mature. It can be used to help one relax and sleep.

6. Obsidian

Obsidian is a type of volcanic glass which has been formed by the action of lava. It is very grounding, and can be used to relieve anxiety, stress, and fears. This type of crystal is also very useful for protection against various kinds of psychic attacks whether they be physical or emotional.

Obsidian can help dispel obsessive thoughts and negative energy, helping one to confront painful situations courageously without running away.

7. Aquamarine

This crystal is used for healing the throat chakra, so it has a special affinity for strengthening the vocal cords and cleansing the thyroid gland which can become inflamed due to constant anger issues or rage attacks.

8. Turquoise

This crystal is one of the most powerful energies in nature because it can call forth the inner child to heal. It brings serenity, trust and tranquility which are all very healing for those who are having difficulties in their lives. This crystal aids those who have had traumatizing events in their lifetime and helps them release these traumas so they can find peace.

9. Excaliburite

This is a type of obsidian which is more purple or bluish gray than black, and it has a purple hue to it as well as gray, white and pink veins running through the crystal. It is considered to be one of the most powerful healing crystals due to its extensive connection with spiritual realms as well as with Mother Earth.

10. Tiger's eye

This is a quartz and one of the most powerful crystals in the healing and spiritual realms. It has strong energy but is also soothing and gentle at the same time. It can help one to see their truth and can clear negative energy, so it is not interfering with life.

11. Black tourmaline

This crystal has a purple hue to it due to its presence of iron (which gives it its dark color). This crystal is useful in opening psychic abilities, reaching spirit entities and healing the heart chakra, which all connect with one's higher self, or God or Goddess.

Common Shapes

Crystals come in different shapes. Among the most common are tumbled stones, which are smooth and rounded, round spheres, and long wands and often cut to resemble a rod. Some have double terminated points at one end, while others have rounded tips.

Another type of shape is the egg-shaped crystal which is oval shaped with pointed ends at both ends rather than just one. These are considered mighty stones because they connect one with the divine feminine energy or Goddess energy. After all, it represents the egg holding within its new life and rebirth after death. After all, it looks very much like an embryo inside its egg-shaped shell. Other common shapes include various types of pyramids. These can be cut into different sizes, from minor to relatively large.

The most common stone used for this purpose is the clear quartz crystal because it is a master healer and acts as a harmonizer within the body and other crystals.

Healing crystals are those that have been polished to a smooth surface free from indentations, cracks, or other imperfections. Any healing stone can be used as a healing stone as long as it is clean and clear of defects. Specific stones are said to attract the energy of the particular element they are associated with. For example, black tourmalines are said to attract all types of fuel, including the fire element.

1. The Pyramid

Crystals of this shape are said to heal all seven chakras. Specific crystals are associated with each chakra. But it is said that if one can't afford to purchase a particular type of stone (e.g., the diamond), then the pyramid is a good substitute since it will still result in healing on all seven chakras. It has been found that the more profound the pyramid, the more power it holds and therefore, if one can afford a deep pyramid, then one should do so since this may give more benefit.

The pyramid connects one to the Earth's energy and links one directly to the Creator. When using a pyramid, one can place or hold a crystal inside it and place this in a location that will get plenty of sunlight, but not too much.

2. The Sphere

These are used to connect one with love and the universal law of attraction. It expands one's vibration, attracts abundance, and makes one feel whole. Holding or wearing a sphere can take away stress and tension; it is perfect for the first chakra since it is associated with creativity, pleasure, and sensuality, all of which promote happiness. Stress depletes our emotional energy; holding a sphere will bring back emotional energy lost due to pressure to where it needs to be.

3. The egg

Egg-shaped crystals are said to be the most potent and most influential of all shapes. People can use them to heal all body parts and even injuries sustained in the womb before it is born. It is very receptive to healing energies, balances one's energy fields, raises one's vibration, helps one become more spiritual. Increases feminine energy-the Goddess energy attracts love into one's life along with abundance, success in career or business. Fertility in general (most often, this will involve conception) and can help with anything related to money.

4. The Crescent

The crescent-shaped crystal is associated with the third eye chakra, which lies between the eyebrows at the center of the foreheads. It is an opening to the spiritual world. The third eye is also associated with intuition, psychic phenomena, clairvoyance, precognition, dream recall.

When using a crescent-shaped crystal, one would hold it between the thumb and first finger of the opposite hand and point it to one's third eye chakra. This connects one to all things that are spiritual or that come from the spirit world.

5. The Geode

According to some crystal healers, umbrella-shaped crystals evoke divine masculine energy, which can help manifest abundance. One should hold the umbrella crystal in one's left palm with both hands cupped together. Point the umbrella handle upward toward the sky. This is a way to connect through prayer and meditation with the divine masculine energy, thanking the Creator for all His blessings and asking for more things that one wants in life.

6. The Pointed Wand

A pointed wand is a good tool for healing because it channels and directs energy very well. One should hold this between both palms and point it toward whatever area of body or aura that is being worked on, directing the healing energies where they need to go.

7. The heart

The heart shape crystal has the ability to balance the entire body and clear away any blockages that may be present within it. To use this crystal, one would hold it between the thumb and forefinger of the opposite hand and point it at the heart. This will activate all chakras. One can hold a crystal in each hand and point them both toward one's own heart to heal all parts of the body.

8. The Hexagram

The hexagram is used to attract abundance and prosperity through meditation, prayer, and intention. It is said to help one find the proper path toward the completion of one's goals in life.

One should hold the hexagram (two triangles, one inverted over the other) with both hands, one pointing upward and the other pointing downward. The point of each triangle should be away from one's body.

Choosing a Crystal

No matter which type of crystal one chooses, it is essential to choose a clear, free from cracks or indents. It should also be bought from a reputable source as there are many fake crystals out there advertised as accurate. When comparing multiple crystals, one should take note of the specific chakras associated with each crystal. Crystals are said to heal through particular chakras. Crystals useful for healing can also be used for other purposes; for example, if one desires to attract abundance into their life, then one could use a hexagram shaped crystal, since it is said to attract a lot.

Some people who practice natural healing (not only using crystals) say that the colour of the crystal does make a difference; however, others say that this is not true—that it's only the shape and size which make the difference. It is said that the red colour of crystals is used to heal physical problems, for example, cancer.

The orange colour is used for curing diseases like arthritis, AIDS, and other immune system-related disorders. The yellow crystals aid in healing lung disorders like bronchitis and emphysema. Blue is used for curing liver diseases or diseases that affect the heart; green is good for cleansing the blood; purple stones are helpful in cases of Alzheimer's disease. Purple can also help with skin disorders like acne.

Multiple Crystals?

Some people have the same crystal for many different purposes. For example, one can have a heart-shaped quartz crystal for healing and attract love and abundance. One can have a citrine crystal for wealth and use it in recovery because citrine is associated with the solar plexus chakra, which is related to benevolent power and abundance.

Someone may wish to have a quartz crystal in an egg shape to be used for both healing and prosperity. It is essential to have a clear idea of your goals beforehand when choosing multiple crystals.

When choosing multiple crystals, keep in mind that they should be held in different positions and with different directions and frequencies. The crystal healer should experiment and note which combinations work best for healing and attracting what one wants.

Some people use multiple crystals simultaneously; for example, one person may use a hexagram crystal for prosperity, while another uses it in healing. If two crystals are used simultaneously, it is essential to make sure that they are sitting inside each other so that they don't spread energy outwards from each other.

Another person may choose to have a crystal in each hand when using them both at once. This is said to be particularly effective. If one is using more than one crystal for healing, it is said that they should not be directly touching one another.

They should be held in the air with an inch or two of space between them. This is important because it keeps the energy within them and doesn't let it escape or become lost, thus creating a weaker and less effective healing session.

Many people might think that it would be wasteful to buy more than one crystal when one could use the same crystal for multiple purposes. Still, some people feel strongly about this and would not want another person's energy within their healing jewel while trying to do healing work with it. Others may choose to use more than one crystal at once.

One can hold two crystals in the palm of their hand while using both at the same time. Another person may put one crystal in each hand or place them around their neck on chains; this increases the power of the healing session by bringing more energy into it.

When choosing more than one crystal, it is essential to remember that they should not touch one another while they are held together. One must also never put them in direct contact with each other (for example, on top of each other). Choosing crystals that are too close to one another will cause an imbalance and unbalance, working against one's healing purposes.

Buyer Beware

To tell authentic crystals from fake ones, it is said that they should be held in front of a light source. Artificial crystal will cast a shadow when held near light; genuine crystal will not cast a shadow, but instead, it will absorb the light and shine brightly with its inner luminescence. Often, fake crystals are also not "clear" like real ones; instead, they are opaque, making them appear like glass with glitter (genuine crystals are clear like window glass).

Scratching a crystal will reveal if it is accurate or fake. Fake crystals tend to be rougher and have a frosty appearance. Natural crystals have a smoother appearance and do not have a frosty appearance.

A final test of whether or not one's crystal is real, or fake is to hold it in front of an open flame. Genuine crystal will not be affected by flames; artificial crystal will be destroyed by it.

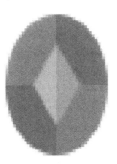

CHAPTER THREE: TAKING CARE OF CRYSTALS

Before you use those healing crystals, how do you cleanse, bless, charge, and program them? What are the basic precautions to take with crystals?

You can call them Angel Stones or Crystal Vaults, regardless of what you call them, these stones are beautiful.

In truth, it is okay to consider a cracked crystal as being beautiful because it speaks of love and healing from within themselves. This chapter will help you understand the use of stones and why they are used for cleansing, chargeing, blessing and programing. It might be interesting that, you don't have to use the whole rock in healing or program them with yourself or others because each stone has its frequency, and it will work for its owner/user.

Cleansing Your Crystals

Cleansing is the art of de-programming the stones. The divine energy in stones vibrates at specific frequencies and does not like to be disturbed. When you cleanse them or charge them, you take away the programming given to these stones, to allow them to work for you. You need to wash your stones before giving or setting them with any other programming or energy.

To cleanse your stones, you need to repeat this process at least three times.

- Take your stone and hold it in your hand and close your eyes and let the energy flow through you. Feel the energy or frequency of this stone and release all thoughts from your mind.

- Now put the crystal back in its holder and take a deep breath, now breathe out

- Repeat this process three times

- After cleansing, charge your stone

Charging Your Crystals

Charging is the process of putting energy into your stone to make it work for you. To charge your stones, you need to take them out of their holder and place them on a clean cloth. Make sure that the crystals are never touching each other while charging or when using them. You can also place crystals directly on the skin if you want to do healing work with them.

- Now, hold your stone in your hand and feel its energy emanating through your body

- Connect with the energy and say, " (name of stone) I am now charging you with the divine energy of (name of God/Divine power)

- Hold your stone in your hand and feel the vibration. This is the energy you are charging

- Repeat this process 2 to 3 times

- You can also charge your stones by putting them on metal (preferably copper) plates and place them on a windowsill. Come back after 20 hours and check if they are charged or not.

- You can also charge your crystals by placing them in direct sunlight or moonlight for a day.

- Remember, you must cleanse the stone before charging it to attract divine energy easier and work with you better.

Programming Your Crystals

Programming is the process of giving an intention to your crystal. This way, when you use them for healing, they will fulfil the purpose for which you had programmed them. To program your stones, take them out of their holder and place them on a clean cloth. Hold the stone in your hand and put it over an organ (like heart chakra) where it is needed most; feel its energy flowing through that body part.

- To program your stones, sit still and concentrate on the rock and ask it to channel its energy to heal the body part. If you are using more than one crystal at a time, place them around your neck and let their energy flow into that area of your body.

- If you want to clear out some negative energy or some blockage in your body, just put the crystals on the affected area and feel it clearing out all negative energies.

- Repeat this process 2 to 3 times

Once you have programmed your stones, keep them in their holder or keep them around your neck (if you had programmed them). These stones will activate themselves when they sense that they need to work for you.

Preparing Your Space

Remember that crystals are energy powerful, and powerful energy needs space to be effective. If you keep your crystals in the same room as they were before, they will lose their effectiveness. To keep them working for you, you need to create a sacred space that is loving and can connect with their energy.

Whenever you want to use your stones, take them out of the holder and place them in a different position in this space.

If you keep your stones in the same room as before, you need to change their position every time you want to use them.

- Keep them on different tables or different corners of the room.

Ensure that there are no electromagnetic fields (like microwave ovens, television sets, computers, power lines, etc.) around them because they will interfere with their effectiveness.

- Keep your stones in a separate space from your computer and other electronic devices so that they can have better energy contact with them. You can also take time out from all electronics for a few hours each day so that the crystals have a chance to connect with their energy without being disturbed by electronics and technology.

Preparing Your Mind

For your crystals to be effective, you must have a positive attitude when working with them. When you are working with your stones, keep in mind that they can help and heal and improve yourself and others with their energies. Do not place them around negative people because the energy will be absorbed by them and will stop your connection with the power of the crystals. You can read up on their points beforehand to know how to use them in a healing way. These energies are generally used for good but can be used negatively.

The quickest way to get rid of bad vibes is to be aware of your surroundings and make sure that you are not in a hostile place while using your crystals. They can still help you no matter how you feel but remember that your mainframe will affect their power to help you. This applies to people who are trying to heal themselves as well. If you are not focused on the healing the crystals are helping to give, it will seem like they are not doing anything. They can also be effective when placed around water because minerals have an energy of their own, which penetrates all matter.

Meditation is a good way of clearing your mind of any negative thoughts and learning to understand the language of the crystals. If you meditate, you can learn to perceive what your crystals are trying to communicate. By doing this, you will be able to determine what they need from you for them to be able to heal you or someone else. With enough practice, however, they will tell you what their own needs are. It is similar to how a doctor determines a course of treatment for a sick person because they can read their pulse and listen to their heartbeat.

Preparing Your Body

When you are going to use a crystal, it is a good idea to ground yourself. The easiest way to do this is to have something that you can touch the ground. You can use a tree, a rock, or even your house if you cannot get outside. In any case, the most crucial part about grounding yourself is that you have something physical that you can connect with for your mind and body to be working in harmony. This will ensure that your energy levels are even and balanced when trying to heal someone in need of help.

It also keeps you from feeling tired and drained if there is a lot of sickness in the area around you.

Please take off your shoes and socks to make sure that you are physically connecting yourself with the energy of the Earth through your crystals. While this may not mean anything to some people, it can be essential to associate yourself with the Earth's power. The soles of your feet have a connection to the ground and can help you maintain balance when working with crystals.

If you want, you can take a walk outside where you live before beginning your healing session. This will help link yourself with nature and make your session more effective. Connect with some dirt or go into another room where there is some dirt, and connect yourself with it for a little while, before sitting down in front of your stones and beginning your session. When you're grounded, the rocks will have a much better effect on you and those you are trying to heal.

One of the most important things you can do is stay away from alcohol and refrain from smoking cigarettes or marijuana before your session begins.

It would be best if you were as clean as possible, for the crystals to transmit their healing powers through you. The more drugs and alcohol you have in your system, the lower the amount of healing will occur during your session.

Handling healing stones

When holding a crystal, make sure that you concentrate on how it feels by using your entire hand. Hold it against your hand and focus on what you feel in your fingers. If, for any reason, you do not feel anything, then move the crystal around in a circle, around the outside of the hand that is holding it.

It is an excellent idea to take a deep breath while doing this so that you can fully appreciate the feeling when it happens. Holding crystals against your skin can help stimulate healing processes because they have been known to release negative ions into the body when in touch with the skin. Proven medical studies have yet to be accepted by all doctors as a legitimate way of improving physical health.

Still, some people find that they are more comfortable being healed by crystals than by modern medicine.

After you have handled your crystals and relaxed, you can begin your healing session. It is a good idea to work together with other people who are also trying to heal themselves with the crystals. The energy will become amplified through everyone in the room, and they will be more successful in helping out those that need it. Be sure that you are not wearing clothes that might absorb or reflect the energy of any of your crystals because they could cause problems when trying to heal people.

Respecting your stones

It is essential to treat your crystals with respect and take care of them when used. Some people like to wrap them up in silk or put them inside a pouch to ensure that they are not getting damaged or chipped. You can also keep them in a special box with only the crystals that are meant for healing. This way, you will not be confused about which crystals you are supposed to use for what purpose.

Be sure that you are wearing the stones that are meant for healing, at all times. You can keep them on your body or use them as pieces of jewelry so long as they are touching your skin. If you have a necklace made out of natural materials, then you might want to consider placing one crystal on it so that it can provide extra support during your day-to-day life.

CHAPTER FOUR: CRYSTAL REMEDIES FOR MIND, HEART & SOUL

Stress, anxiety, loneliness, anger, denial, lack of creativity, & confusion—all these negative emotions can affect your energy. When we're unbalanced, it can show up in our lives with a cold, self-pity, or a lot of stress. Crystals are an alternative energy source and can be used to energize your home, stimulate creativity, attract positive people & money into your life.

Have you ever realized that when you are feeling down, you can put on a crystal necklace, one with a quartz point in it, and instantly feel better? Like someone has pinched your energy. Then put on an amethyst or citrine or any stone with beautiful cathedral-window-style crystals in it. Crystals are the ultimate cure for negative thoughts & feelings. They open up your heart & mind to feel connected with the world around you.

How to balance the chakras with healing stones

Each of the seven chakras is a spiritual center in the human body, and each has a unique energy system that influences mental and physical health. The chakras affect electrical energy in the body, called the "life force," over which we have some degree of control. The heart chakra, for example, is considered our second brain because it's located close to the throat chakra. It's where conscious & unconscious thoughts or feelings are communicated from one to another or from our inner self to our environment.

Crystal healing involves placing crystals on each of the seven major chakras of your body for a quick cure-all treatment. Each crystal can be used for more than one purpose while you're going through different life changes.

To balance the crown chakra, where you are most spiritually evolved, clear away all unnecessary clutter in your life. Get rid of all the junk you've accumulated over the years. Even if you want to keep it, choose wisely. If it's an out-of-date shirt, your mother gave you, toss it or give it to a friend or relative. If you have an extra sweater at home that's too big for you, donate to a thrift store or recycle it for new clothing for some other person in poverty. Don't hoard things that don't bring any healing energy into your life.

When you're done clearing out your space, put an accountability crystal there in the crown chakra. Be careful in this area not to pick any quartz crystals that are too old or have been in contact with alcohol or chemicals. You can cleanse Quartz by placing it into a bowl of water with some sea salt, then set the bowl next to it on your altar or your bedside table, and let the crystals run their energy through each other. If you want to boost your power, place a long-standing crystal on your crown chakra.

For energy and creativity, you'll want to put a rose crystal on your altar or your bedside table. The rose quartz is the perfect crystal for creative energy because it's romantic and gives you a boost of confidence, and it's a deep pink colour, fitting for the crown chakra.

Rose quartz has been worn and used for centuries and has proven effective in many diseases, from headaches to rheumatism to blood problems. You can also use a crystal pendulum or a particular "crystal ball" showing you what your future holds.

The throat chakra is where we communicate with our environment and our inner selves as survival instincts arise from within us. Use an amethyst or citrine crystal here to balance your energy. It will stop you from speaking words that are harmful to your life.

Amethyst is a very effective crystal for healing any throat disease, but it inhibits the transmission of nerve impulses between the brain & spinal column. Citrine can heal inflammation of the vocal cords & swelling, as well as rheumatism, arthritis, & diseases of lymph glands. They're both effective at clearing sinuses; also affects metabolism (helps your body metabolize food).

To relieve fears or misfortunes that affect our speech flow, like stuttering or laryngitis (which affects 2 million Americans), this crystal on your throat chakra will help you speak clearly & promote good vocal health.

This crystal also balances the nervous system, which is part of your life force energy system.

The solar plexus chakra is where we store our feelings & emotions. Use an amethyst or citrine crystal here to balance your feelings & emotions, giving you the confidence to act upon them.

Amethyst is used for regulating the nervous system because it can heal nerve disorders caused by stress or nervousness. Citrine balances all the other crystals in the chakra by removing any blockages that could affect your speech or creativity. It reduces stress and anxiety, making it very helpful to focus on a problem or accomplish a goal.

Manifesting money, wealth and abundance

Think of a time you wanted something so badly, and the universe gave it to you. It could be as simple as a parking spot at the mall or as big as winning £10 million in the lottery. When you want something badly enough and give it enough life force energy, it'll show up one way or another. So how do we create positive energy that attracts good things to us? Think of the universe as your creative energy source & imagine what you can do with that creative energy.

You can create a bigger home, a new car, a more extensive bank account.

Crystals can help you let go of negative energy & attract positive energy. When you create your positive energy, you'll be willing to accept the beautiful things the universe has in store for you. That's why clearing out negative feelings is very important for manifesting good things in your life. It all begins with healing crystals from each of the seven major chakras.

The money chakra is located just below your belly button and affects your self-image and how other people see & treat you as well as how much money and resources you attract into your life.

To improve your self-image, put a golden tiger's eye crystal in this chakra. The tiger's eye makes you feel more attractive & confident about who you are. For easy access to naturally attract money into your life, keep a pebble of onyx near the area where dollars come in.

The law of attraction involves being positive in your thoughts & actions to attract prosperity, health, love & happiness into your life. But there are times when you have to be realistic about money matters.

You can't just think about how much money you want & expect the universe to give it to you. You have to be realistic in your thinking so that the universe knows exactly what it's doing with all that positive energy.

This crystal is ideal for the heart chakra because it promotes selfless love & compassion, keeping your heart open & allowing outside energies in to make some severe changes in your life. The fluorite crystal will pick up on some of the negative aspects of the heart chakra, like anger, resentment or jealousy.

Using crystals to manifest love

Romantic relationships are something most of us dream about & living in a world full of love is something we all crave. But when it doesn't happen, the heart chakra can feel empty & lonesome. It can lead to negativity or disillusionment when the person you're in love with doesn't feel the same way about you.

Bring a beautiful rose quartz crystal into your life to help fill your heart chakra with positive energy.

Rose quartz is one of the most popular crystals used in healing, but it's essential that rose quartz has not been exposed to air, toxins, or chemicals. It's like a self-cleaning oven; it cleanses itself of any negative energy & will transform into clear Quartz or diamond.

Rose quartz is ideal for the heart chakra because it balances your emotions, making you calmer & love. It's also good for relieving fear and stress and cleanses the aura of negative energies. When you surround yourself with rose quartz, you'll feel happiness and contentment in your life.

Using crystals to improve reproductive health

If you are trying to conceive, chances are you've got many questions about your body & how it works. Chances are you may even have some dreams about the baby you haven't given birth to yet. To help conceive a healthy child, use one of the crystal healings stones that are good for conception &/or pregnancy.

The amethyst crystal is excellent for balancing hormones in pregnancy, which can influence the development of the all-important yolk sac & placenta for a healthy birth.

The onyx stone opens up blocked or recessed energy in the body, making it easier for reproductive organs to work correctly and keep track of fertility. Imbalanced hormones can affect all parts of the reproductive system, including ovaries & testicles, the uterus, clitoris & the womb. One of the ways onyxes strengthens your immune system is by encouraging circulation in your reproductive organs.

Chakra healing for heart problems

Heart disease is the number one killer of women worldwide: it's also one of the most common causes of death in men. Heart health is essential because it affects our overall health & longevity.

Heart chakra stones are beneficial when dealing with issues that might cause an irregular heartbeat or high blood pressure, like anxiety disorders or depression. The heart crystal will help you realize your true self, to feel good about yourself & bring peace to your life.

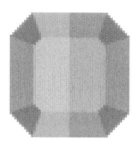

CHAPTER FIVE: CRYSTAL REMEDIES FOR OVERLAPPING AREAS

Addiction & Self-Control

Gluttony, overindulging in alcohol or drugs, smoking, shopping, or gambling could all be signs of an addiction. If you feel like your life is out of control & you can't stop yourself from doing certain things despite adverse consequences, it might be time to work on your self-control & discipline.

Crystal healing can help improve self-control because it's like a form of psychotherapy. Using the healing properties of crystals, helps eliminate negative thoughts and behaviour and replace them with positive ones. Crystals can also help those who've struggled with drug or alcohol addiction for years, find the strength to quit & stay clean by reminding them to make better choices for their future.

Sobriety Crystals like green jasper, rhodonite, or moss agate can help with self-control because they can help you stop overindulging if you're the type who has to eat one more piece of chocolate cake. For people who use crystal meth every day, jasper is a good choice because it helps with motivation. It also helps speedy recovery from withdrawals & mood swings. Self-control is significant for those who want to stay clean, so go ahead & burn some ley line oil for extra protection.

Addiction is a disease, and like all diseases, it will need to be treated like one. Crystal healing can help by bringing you one step closer to recovery.

By giving up drinking or drug abuse, you'll

start developing a healthier mindset that will help you make better decisions in the future. Denial is a crucial part of addiction, and therefore crystal healing can help remove dependence by helping you see the effects of drinking and drug use.

Crystal healing could also teach others about the dangers of addiction & how they might be able to help their loved ones. Helping prevent addiction in others also helps to improve self-control when dealing with habits in your own life.

Anxiety

An anxiety disorder or phobia is a mental health issue that can immobilize you and keep you from doing the daily activities you'd normally do. Social anxiety, obsessive-compulsive disorder (OCD), panic attacks and even post-traumatic stress can all be symptoms of an anxiety disorder. These disorders all have similar symptoms: fear, anxious feelings, shortness of breath, muscle tension, and night sweats.

You may feel crystal healing will only help with symptoms such as insomnia & hot flashes, but it can also help with symptoms such as recurring thoughts, about your illness or fear that something terrible might happen.

Carnelian is one of the most potent crystals for dealing with your fears. Carnelian is said to help you confront your fears & change your behaviour in much the same way that diet & exercise can. This is helpful in cases where you might avoid places or people due to fear or be afraid of future attacks. The redirection of energy helps prevent crisis-level panic attacks & separation anxiety.

Another powerful crystal that can help with anxiety is aquamarine. When paired with another stone-like moonstone, it creates solid spiritual protection for anyone who suffers from fear & who must deal with traumatic events. It could also help those who are afraid of the dark or unsettling things happening.

Depression

Depression is a severe mood disorder affecting millions worldwide each year. Crystals have been used throughout history for their healing properties, but they can also be used for everyday maintenance by helping to bring balance to both the mind & body. If you're feeling low because of low self-esteem or just feeling empty inside, you might want to try crystal healing to improve your attitude toward life & brighten your mood.

Emerald is said to provide a sense of well-being & clarity, which helps you make better choices. It can help support those who are recovering from depression. However, it should only be used by those who are already in treatment for the illness. Emerald can also help relieve stress & lift depression which is often caused by stress or other conditions.

<u>Negativity and catastrophizing</u>

Catastrophizing is when you put the worst possible case scenario in your head and it affects your ability to enjoy life.

If you think something terrible is going to happen or you're faced with a difficult situation, crystal healing can be used to help.

Goji berries and rose quartz are powerful crystals for helping with catastrophizing because they both calm the mind & body. They're also easy to find in nature, making them easy to use in almost any environment or setting. Negativity & catastrophizing can also be caused by living in a negative mindset which is often created by adverse effects of other crystals, such as poorly designed crystals or ones that have been badly cut.

Fear and paranoia are powerful emotions & by putting them in the hands of someone else, you can be in an entirely new situation.

Shyness

Shy people often feel awkward in social situations & overthink what they're supposed to say next when they're trying to make new friends.

They need to work on being themselves, instead of worrying about what others think or what they might say about them.

If you want to deal with shyness, crystal healing is a great way to begin with, because it's self-empowering & requires minimal effort on your part. Lack of confidence can also be caused by low self-esteem, bullying or other trauma in your past. Crystals like tiger iron help with confidence because it helps you speak your mind & helps you to become comfortable with yourself. It's said to give you the strength to know what's right & what's wrong, which is essential for individuals who wants to stand up for themselves or others.

Procrastination

You're living in an age where everyone has the latest technology at their fingertips, keeping up could be causing you anxiety. If you're not sure how to handle all this new information, then it might be causing stress that makes focusing on other things difficult. It could also make you feel like you're behind in life & not living up to your potential.

Procrastination can be caused by a lack of motivation or self-discipline, making it difficult to get things done.

If you're looking to eliminate procrastination, crystal healing is an excellent option because it will help to bring the focus back into your life. This is a necessary step for anyone who has trouble getting the things they want done, because it will require effort from you and other people around you.

Crystal healing can help make good choices in life by helping you see other people's perspectives & how their choices will affect them or someone else. When we have too much on our plate, it's hard to take things in one at a time, making us more likely to get overwhelmed & procrastinate.

Quartz is the most powerful crystal to help you get through your daily tasks because it will help you get started on projects right away.

Fear of Failure

Fear of failure is one of the worst fears because it can prevent you from doing anything at all. You might be worried about failing & not living up to expectations which may cause you to do nothing or make rash decisions, in hope that someone will see how hard you're trying. If you're afraid of failure, crystal healing can help.

Quartz is known for bringing abundance into your life which is essential for anyone who wants to succeed. It will also help bring peace of mind & stability, which is crucial to staying on task & getting things done without worrying too much about the outcome.

Guardian angel crystals are good for helping with stress, fears & negative energy, which will make it easier to deal with possible failures in your future. You can also choose crystals that reflect how you would like to live your life, like citrine, fluorite, tiger iron or even Amethyst.

Resentment & Letting Go

Grief & resentment are common emotions that come with loss. Resentment can cause us to hold onto something that was in the past & never forget. If you're holding onto this resentment, it could be causing you to be unhappy or bitter, making it difficult for others to enjoy their lives when they're around you.

If you've lost someone close to you & if your relationship with them ended severely, crystal healing could help you move on by opening your heart back up so that new connections can develop in your life. Letting go of bad relationships is difficult, but if they were the cause of adverse events in your life, it's essential to remove all their reminders so that your life can improve.

Guardian angel stones are suitable for letting go of people & situations that caused you pain in the past. You can also add crystals that reflect how you would like to live your life, like Amethyst, citrine, Quartz, fluorite or even rose Quartz.

Impatience

There's always a lot going on when you're running a business & if you're frustrated by the lack of progress, it could be because it's frustrating to have expectations, about how anything specific should be done, in a certain way. Crystal healing can help resolve this situation because it balances energy so you can allow time to heal any problems without being impatient.

Denial & fear can also be causing you to experience impatience because you're choosing to ignore problems that need to be dealt with. Denial will only make the situation worse, while fear will make it harder for you to get started on a solution.

Crystal healing can help with balancing energy so that you don't have any negative emotions weighing on your mind, which will make it easier to deal with problems & find solutions. You can also protect yourself from what's causing you frustration by wearing crystals like Amethyst, citrine, rose Quartz or clear Quartz.

Lack of Energy

Your life may be full of activity, but if your body needs more sleep, then nothing will work no matter how hard you try. It can be challenging to rest while you're doing something new in your life because you're afraid to stop what you're doing & go to bed. If you're dealing with a lack of energy, crystal healing is a great way to begin with, because it will help you get what you need. You can also put quartz stone under your pillow to bring restful sleep into your life.

CHAPTER SIX: THE SCIENCE & ORIGIN OF CRYSTALS, CHAKRAS & PROPERTIES

Actinolite

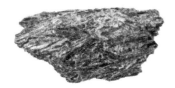

The amphibole silicate mineral that crystallizes has long blades or a thin needle-like structure. This crystal is most commonly found in its distinctive dark green colour, but it can also be white, yellow, grey, or black. R. Kirwan was the first to record this mineral in 1794. He named it "Aktis," which means "beam or ray" in Greek. To describe the shape of Actinolite, and the name has stuck since then. Actinolite is a relatively common crystal that can be found all over the world. Brazil, Russia, Canada, China, and the United States all have an abundance of this mineral beneath their feet!

Chakras for the heart

Properties

Resolution, Joy, Knowledge

Love & Relationships, Meditation

New Beginnings, Nourishing and Rejuvenation

Nurturing, Peace of Mind, Physical Healing

Relaxation, Intuition, Self- Healing

Self-Discovery, Selflessness, Soothing

Stress Relief, Trust, Truth, Creating Your Own Reality

Anxiety Relief, Calming and Patience

Claiming Wholeness, Compassion

Consciousness

Aquamarine

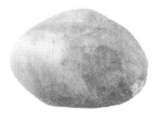

Aquamarine is a blue Beryl crystallization that forms hexagonal columns. Trace amounts of iron cause the blue colour of this stone, frequently found in conjunction with Muscovite. This mineral was first used around 400 B.C. in Greece, but multiple societies have used it for over 2,000 years. Aquamarine can be found in the United States, Brazil, Australia, and several other African countries. Pakistan and Afghanistan are currently producing the highest quality specimens on the market.

Chakras for the throat and heart

<u>Properties</u>

Anger & Stress

Energy/Rejuvenation, Calming and Patience

Inspiration, Protection

Higher Self, Insight

Expanded Awareness, Inner Peace

Peace of Mind, Anxiety Relief

Black Opal

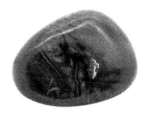

Black Opal is a sheer variety of Popular Opal. The above variation is most commonly found in mass form and is a trendy material to cut into palm stones, carvings, and jewellery. Other colours, including brown, white, grey, and beige, can be found in sizeable Black Opal specimens even though Australia is known to have an abundance of this mineral. A few of the most delicate pieces of Black Opal have been extracted from Oregon.

Chakras for the root

<u>Properties</u>

Creating Your Own Reality, Enlightenment

Stress Relief, Soothing, Resolution

Relaxation, Protection, Peace of Mind

Meditation, Inner Peace, Empathy

Emotional Understanding

Compassion, Claiming Wholeness

Calming and Patience, Anxiety Relief

Blue Topaz

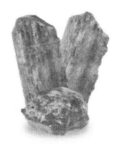

Blue Topaz, a unique variety of Topaz, is an aluminium fluorine silicate mineral that forms in relatively small (well-formed) vertical hexagonal crystals and tiny prismatic shards. The colours are produced by unstable light that is directly absorbed by the iron atom aggregates. Texas' state mineral seems to be blue Topaz, and small deposits have been discovered. Latin America and Zimbabwe are the most commercialized countries.

Chakras for the third Eye and throat

<u>Properties</u>

Relaxation, Inner Peace, Inner Vision

Insight, Inspiration

Interdimensional Communication

Intuition, Knowledge

Living in the Present Moment

Mental Enhancement, Peace of Mind

Psychic Abilities, PTSD

Higher Self, Resolution

Self-Discipline, Self- Healing

Self-Discovery, Selflessness

Carnelian

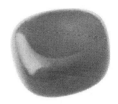

Carnelian is a popular member of the Quartz family and is an orange/reddish variety of Smoky Quartz (but can also be found nearly all black). It is derived from the mediaeval Latin word Corneolus, which refers to the Cornelian cherry, a plant native to southern Europe. Carnelian can be found all over the world, as civilizations throughout history have demonstrated! The majority of Carnelian specimens on the market are from Brazil, Uruguay, Madagascar, and India.

Chakras for the Solar Plexus, Sacral and Root

<u>Properties</u>

Strength, Courage

Confidence, Power

Grounding

Passion, Manifestation

Action

Sexuality, Motivation

Citrine

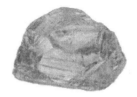

Citrine is the name given to a yellowish/orange variety of Quartz that contains Iron elements. It can be crystallized in just about any form that Quartz can be found. Its name is derivative of the Greek word, which translates to Citron. Citrine from the Minas Geras region of Brazil is the most famous in the world, followed by Sri Lanka and India. Beautiful specimens have recently been discovered in Madagascar. This crystal, on the other hand, can be found almost anywhere.

Chakras for the Third Eye, Solar Plexus, Sacral and Root

Properties

Inspiration, Dreams, Joy

Transmutation of Negative Energies

Creativity, Clarity, Protection

Abundance, Manifestation

Weight Control, Personal Will

Anxiety Relief, Balancing Polarities

Strength

Hematite

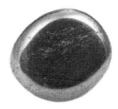

Hematite is a common iron oxide, natural substance, botryoidal, tabular. The rarest form of rhombohedral crystals. This mineral, which was initially known as "Haematite," was not officially discovered until 1773 by Jean Baptiste Rome de I'Isle, who removed the first "e" to make it "Hematite." The mineral's name comes from the Greek word for blood, "haima," simply because of the colour it takes when ground to powder. Hematite is a rare mineral that was thought to have been used by humans 164,000 years ago.

Chakras for the Root

Properties

Opportunities

Strength, Balance, Clarity, Meditation

Grounding, Focus, Alignment of Chakra

Balancing Polarities, Manifestation

Action, Mental Enhancement

Howlite

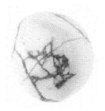

Howlite, also recognized as Magnesite, is a calcium borosilicate hydroxide mineral that crystallizes as masses, nodules, and rare tiny prismatic crystals. It's most commonly seen in a colour scheme of chalky white with black veins running through it. It can, however, be perceived as brown or even colourless. Howlite was discovered near Windsor, Nova Scotia, in 1868.

Chakras for the Crown

Properties

Calming and Patience, Strength

Balance, Creativity, Inspiration

Confidence, Knowledge, Physical Healing

Atonement, Truth, Consciousness

Stress Relief

Himalayan Quartz

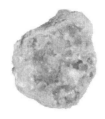

Himalayan Quartz is a rare but rather ancient type of Quartz that was established in the Himalayan Mountains. This mountain range connects Nepal and Bhutan, as well as forming the boundary between India and China. These one-of-a-kind crystals can develop in various sizes and shapes, including prismatic, tabular, clusters, and skinny needle-like points. Since some of the matrices it forms on are brittle enough to break in your hand, this Quartz variety is exceptionally fragile.

Chakras for the Crown, Third Eye, throat, heart, Solar Plexus, Sacral and Root

Properties

Calming and Patience, Psychic Abilities

Joy, Balance, Opportunities, Intuition

Inspiration, Clarity, Transformation

Meditation, Courage, Confidence

Knowledge, Power, Synchronicity

Physical Healing, Empathy, Channelling

Grounding, Purification, Atonement

Clairvoyance, Ascension, Truth

Self-Discipline, Altruism, Consciousness

Leadership, Relaxation

Rose Quartz

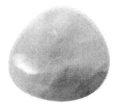

Rose Quartz is among the most common types in the Quartz family, and it is found mainly in Brazil, Madagascar, and South Dakota (USA). It usually forms in the cores of granite pegmatites and also has a hazy to semi-transparent appearance. Its colour ranges from light pale pink to deep hot pink (with reddish undertones) and is caused by trace amounts of titanium, iron, and manganese. The colour is very stable and will not fade when exposed to heat or natural sun.

Chakras for the heart

<u>Properties</u>

Self-Love, Soothing,

Calming and Patience

Love & Relationships, Joy,

Creativity

Clearing, Physical Healing,

Empathy, Cleansing, Relaxation,

Anxiety Relief

Sapphire

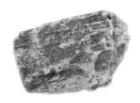

Sapphire is a type of corundum that was discovered in 1747 by J.G. Wallerius. He named the stone "Sapphires," which means "blue stone," about the mineral's colour. Despite being reported in 1747, sapphire has also been traced back to the ancient Romans 3000 bc. Sapphire has also been regarded as a royal stone by the civilizations of Ancient Greece and Egypt.

Chakras for the Crown, Third Eye, throat, heart, Solar Plexus, Sacral and Root

Properties

High Vibration, Psychic Abilities

Strength, Love & Relationships

Creativity, Transformation

Communication, Protection

Self-Discipline, Higher Self

Abundance, Prosperity

Gentle Self-Expression

Expanded Awareness

Turquoise

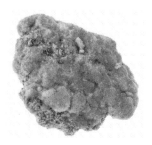

Turquoise is a natural component of copper and aluminium. Copper causes the bright blue colour, and the greenish hues are caused by iron speckles within. It got its name from the French "Pierre turquoise," which means "Turkish stone," even though Turkey traded a lot of turquoise because of its location between Europe and Asia. Turquoise is one of, if not the, oldest stones in human history.

Chakras for the throat

Properties

Travel, Balance

Communication, Empathy

Truth, Stress Relief, Higher Self

Expansion, Expanded Awareness

Inner Peace, Self-Healing

Peace of Mind

Emotional Understanding

CHAPTER SEVEN: CRYSTALS COME IN MANY FORMS

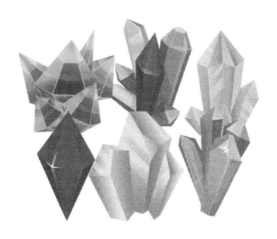

Beads of prayer

Crystal prayer beads are worn against the heart to evoke positive emotions such as hope, courage, and peace. They're an excellent way for anyone to carry the healing powers of crystals with them.

Crystal embellishments

The main advantage of crystals may be their healing properties. But, if we're being completely honest, they're also quite lovely. As a result, it's no surprise that they're used to make a variety of accessories, such as jewelry and home decorations.

Not only will the crystals look nice but having positive energy around will never hurt anyone.

Bottles of water

Water bottles are often just as fashionable as crystals these days, so it's no surprise that the two have been combined. A "gem container" sinks to the bottom of these lovely cans and bottles.
It is said to promote everything from health and beauty products to balance. This is an excellent addition to your next yoga practice.

Coasters

These stunning coasters are made from genuine Brazilian gemstones. This product's agate rock will help to promote harmony and balance in the home. These are ideal for people who want to bring positive energy into their home.

Pipes

Whether you believe it or not, you can smoke from crystal-made hand pipes. They're smooth, simple to use, and durable. As a result, they make an excellent gift for anyone who uses medical marijuana to treat a medical condition.

Jewelry

Jewelry is another excellent way to introduce a crystal's abilities. To recognize that it allows you to highlight the beauty of each stone.

Sex Toys

These crystal toys for sex combine their energies with your sexual energy to aid in the delivery of pure sexual pleasure. They're excellent tools for those who have been stuck in sexual doldrums and want to break free.

Technology

Quartz crystals have a natural exposure to piezoelectricity, which allows them to generate an electrical field, making them extremely useful in radio and video equipment. Silicon crystals are used for the manufacture of computer chips as well as photovoltaic panels used in renewable technology. Crystals are often cut and polished into gemstones used in jewelry. Crystals are frequently used as decorative items as well as focal points in meditation and healing practices.

CHAPTER EIGHT: IS THERE SUCH THING AS WITCHCRAFT USING CRYSTALS?

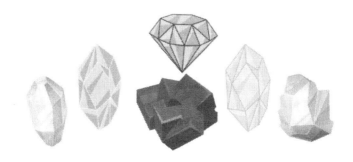

As well as being used for its beauty, crystals and gemstones have also been used for witchcraft. Though all witchcraft is not always evil, many would link witchcraft to negativity, such as casting spells that might be considered hurtful. Such as Love, Revenge, Money, and good luck spells.

There are many professional psychics and witches out there with backed up claims to tap into specific energies and redirect that energy on your behalf.

Quite frankly, this is not an area of concentration to the author; she is somewhat a misanthropist when it comes to using crystals to practice witchcraft and whether it works as a result, or just coincidental. It is important to note that psychics and witches use crystals differently.

Wicca & Witchcraft

Witch doctors use Crystals in the art of practicing Wicca & Witchcraft; crystals are said to have the power to move the energy in and around a person or situation.

Wicca

A predominantly Western movement whose followers practice witchcraft and nature worship and see it as a religion based on the pre-Christian traditions of northern and western Europe. It spread across England in the 1950s and later attracted a following in Europe and the United States.

Witchcraft

Someone who practices witchcraft communicate with the devil or with a familiar person or thing and or the use of sorcery or magic.

Crystals are an essential tool in a witch's magical practices. I love crystals because they are stunning. In addition, each one has its unique properties. It's like each crystal has its very own unique character and energy.

Though the use of crystals for witchcraft is a specialist topic, this book will include some information that beginners and seasoned witches may find thought-provoking.

Many witches are associated with at least one stone. It's generally a direct connection they experience undoubtedly with their energies.
Some relate to howlite, predominantly white, which helps with sleep problems, or rose Quartz, for its loving energy.

The most popular crystals for witches

Rose quartz, Clear Quartz and Black obsidian are the best crystals for witches, though there are many other choices on the market.

Clear Quartz

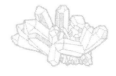

This is one of the essential crystals to have in your arsenal of pretty rocks. It can be used to not only amplify the energies of surrounding crystals, but clear Quartz can also replace any crystal you need in a spell or ritual.

This is one of the highly vital crystals to have in your collection of rocks. The most effective in its uses is to expand the energies of the encompassing crystals; however, the vibrant Quartz can also be substituted for any crystal you want in a spell or ritual.

Rose Quartz

You are known as the "mother stone" and the stone of universal love. This pink stone makes you feel love when you hold it in your hand. Rose quartz cleanses and opens the heart on all levels to promote love, self-love, friendship, deep inner healing, and feelings of peace. Restores trust and harmony in relationships and encourages unconditional love—also an excellent stone for kids.

This stone is also very easy to find and purchase online or at any store that sells jewelry.

Obsidian

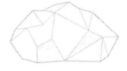

This uniquely simple lava rock known as the black obsidian stone is astonishing for protection and grounding. It can be placed inside your personal belongings for security, such as your bag; it also helps with clarity and has brilliant healing properties; this lava stone can be found anywhere jewelry is sold.

Witches also use the following crystals in their practices.

Amethyst

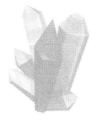

The protective stone is what Amethyst is known for, especially when it comes to harmful behaviours. The ancient Greeks used this purple crystal as an ornament to protect and soothe from getting minor illnesses. Amethyst stone can be found anywhere jewelry is sold.

Lapis Lazuli

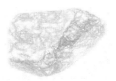

This crystal has a powerful energy. It shields negative vibes, and when used before bed, it can bring vivid dreams of other lives and connections to soulmates who may not be born again at that time.

The main effect of this beautiful blue stone is that you can use it to bring inner knowledge of the other worlds to your mind. If you want to improve your psychic abilities, you must wear this crystal-like form of jewelry all the time.

Psychic

Whenever it comes to interacting with and developing psychic abilities, crystals are used in various ways. Their natural energies can be incorporated into and used to improve skills like divination, scrying, intuition, mediumship, and telepathy. They can be used to hone these abilities as well as to perform readings and other psychic-based work.

Meditation

Crystals can be a significant addition to meditation sessions, developing one's skills while also benefiting and providing insight into all parts of life. Meditation can also assist you in creating a strong bond with and understanding of your crystals. The bonds that can form between you and your crystals are one-of-a-kind and can help ensure that every application is used is successful.

CHAPTER NINE: CAN CRYSTALS ENHANCE PSYHIC ABILITIES

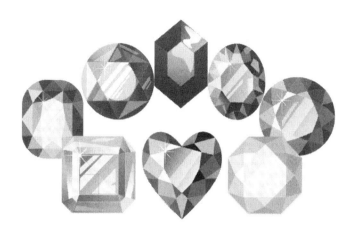

Channelling

Calcite, Agate, and amethyst stones are all thought to be excellent stones for establishing channelling abilities. Keep Amethyst away from your bed, as its ability can indeed cause restless sleep. Calcite and Agate can help you communicate with your guardian angels, while Angelite can help you communicate with spirits.

Clairvoyance

Charoite, apophyllite, and fire agate are all crystals that can assist the reader in seeing the world clearly in the past, present, and future.

Emerald and labradorite crystals are also known to aid clairvoyance.

Clairsentience

Moldavite can help to improve your ability to detect and feel the energies around you.

Astrology

Sphene could help create both a connection to and understanding of both the stars and planets. It will also help you understand how these affect our lives and moods.

Intuition

Charoite, opal, moonstone, rhodolite, sapphire, and tiger's eye are valuable crystals for developing intuition and making sense of the information you receive, even if you don't know where it came from.

Premonition

Opal and prehnite can aid in the development of prophetic visions and dreams.

Crystals that can be used for protection include Agate, aquamarine, lapis lazuli, Smokey Quartz, tiger's eye, and turquoise.

Blue Quartz can aid in the proper interpretation of tarot cards.

Angelite, Blue Quartz, and chalcedony are believed to enhance the capacity to transfer thoughts to others.

Divination

Golden calcite, opal and blue obsidian can all be used to enhance divination. Many crystals have traditional meanings and can be used as part of a divination set.

The crystal types and meaning for divination are as follows

- ❖ Red Jasper- Pay attention to earthy matters.

- ❖ Black agate- You need and will find courage. Prosperity.

- ❖ Aventurine- Further growth and expansion is possible.

- ❖ Garnet- You will soon receive a letter, information or confirmation.

- ❖ Jade- A need for perfection.

- ❖ Citrine- Celestial wisdom will advise you.

- ❖ Clear Quartz- Permanence and advancement. Be sure to clarify issues.

- ❖ Agate- Success or a pleasant surprise. A luck stone for anyone who works with the land. Good health, wealth and a long life.

- ❖ Blue lace agate- Healing is needed.

❖ Red agate- A long and happy life.

❖ Bloodstone- Possibly illness or unwelcome surprise.

❖ Emerald- Fertility.

❖ Hematite- New opportunities are waiting for you.

❖ Lapis lazuli- Luck is in your favour.

❖ Aventurine- Further growth and expansion is possible.

❖ Rose quartz- Self-love and healing are needed and will come in time.

CHAPTER TEN: PUTTING IT ALL TOGETHER

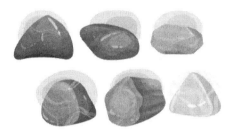

The world is full of fascinating rocks, minerals, gems and even water that have healing properties. They can even be used to heal injuries that were caused by someone else. If you're tired of living in pain, it's time to make the change you need in your life for a more fulfilling life. Crystals are all around us & they can help you overcome adversities when you need them most.

Crystal healing is gaining popularity because it has been proven to work with thousands of people worldwide who are experiencing difficult emotions in their lives. If you're looking for answers in your life, crystal healing may bring peace into your mind, which will open up new opportunities & help you find value in everything that happens in your life.

From what I have discovered, the above crystals are a must-have, when practicing Wicca or Witchcraft, they frequently use most of the stones mention in this book. It is essential to highlight that these stones are beautiful nonetheless, and even though you do not practice Wicca or Witchcraft, it is always handy to own a few of these beautiful precious gems.

Many people have been gifted these pretty little rocks. However, it is handy to know what they are and their many benefits.

If you're already highly skeptical of healing crystals, they're unlikely to help you. Nonetheless, they're unlikely to cause you any harm. However, while there is no scientific evidence for crystals, that hasn't stopped people from trying them.

An attitude of openness is essential for realizing the benefits that these lovely stones could provide. Whether you're looking for good overall energy or specific healing abilities, there's nothing wrong with giving crystals a legitimate chance. Who knows, you might be surprised and delighted.

I hope you have found this topic fascinating; you should have a better understanding of the beautiful power of Crystals, their healing techniques, and how they can be used correctly to benefit you, when considering the seven chakras for the heart, throat and more.

Overall, I hope you have gained the knowledge to choose genuine crystals that can benefit your mind, body & spirit.

ATTRIBUTION

Icons made by [Freepik](www.flaticon.com) from www.flaticon.com

REFERENCE

Aquamarine Meanings and Crystal Properties - The Crystal ....
https://thecrystalcouncil.com/crystals/aquamarine

Carnelian – LuNatura Crystals.
https://lunaturacrystals.com/collections/carnelian

Crystals by Zodiac Sign — The Best Crystals for Each ....
https://www.apartmenttherapy.com/crystals-by-zodiac-sign-36918699

Including Crystals into Your Daily Routine.
https://www.gemexi.com/blog/gemology/including-crystals-into-your-daily-routine

Manifestation Crystal Candles - Casting Candles.
https://castingcandles.com/

How To Use Mindfulness To Stop Procrastinating - Mind Owl. https://mindowl.org/mindfulness-to-stop-procrastinating/

How to Improve Your Life With Positive Energy Stones. https://cosmiccuts.com/blogs/healing-stones-blog/how-to-improve-your-life-with-positive-energy-stones

Rose Quartz Meanings and Crystal Properties - The Crystal .... https://thecrystalcouncil.com/crystals/rose-quartz

https://medium.com/human-witch/the-importance-of-crystals-for-the-baby-witch-2768627f13bf

https://exemplore.com/paranormal/How-to-Use-Crystals-to-Enhance-Psychic-Abilities

A NOTE FROM THE AUTHOR

Thank you so much for choosing to read ***Crystal & Gemstones***.
I hope you enjoyed reading this book as much as I enjoyed writing it. I also hope that you have found this topic useful, and now feel confident when purchasing your beautiful crystals and gemstones that will benefit you personally.

I would like to say a huge thank you to all who have assisted me with the writing of this book, particularly my family and anyone that had an input in the creation of this book.

Reviews are extremely important to authors especially newcomers like me. If you could kindly spend a couple minutes to write an honest review. I would be forever grateful.

Please keep an eye out for new releases and updates via email - info@nimphleebooks.co.uk or Instagram –

NIMPHLEEBOOKS

Thank you
N. Jeffrey

Printed in Great Britain
by Amazon